NO THANK YOU I'M ALLERGIC

A STORY ABOUT FOOD ALLERGY AWARENESS

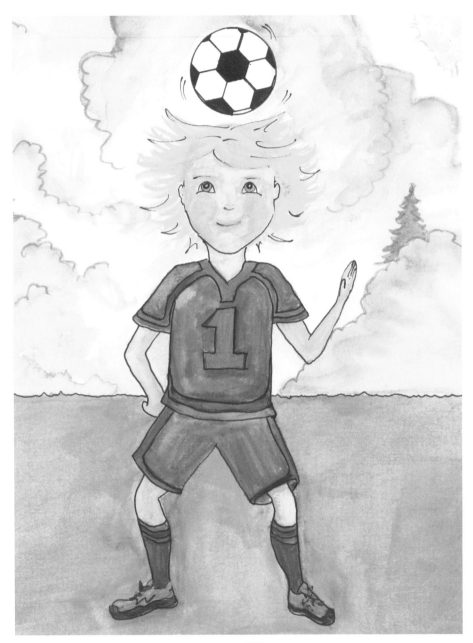

KRISTEN SEYMOUR

ILLUSTRATED BY JAIME STRAUSS

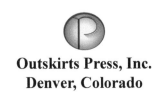

Outskirts Press, Inc.
Denver, Colorado

No Thank You, I'm Allergic
A story about food allergy awareness

Outskirts Press, Inc.
http://www.outskirtspress.com

ISBN: 978-1-4327-3293-6

PRINTED IN THE UNITED STATES OF AMERICA

This Book Belongs to:

_____

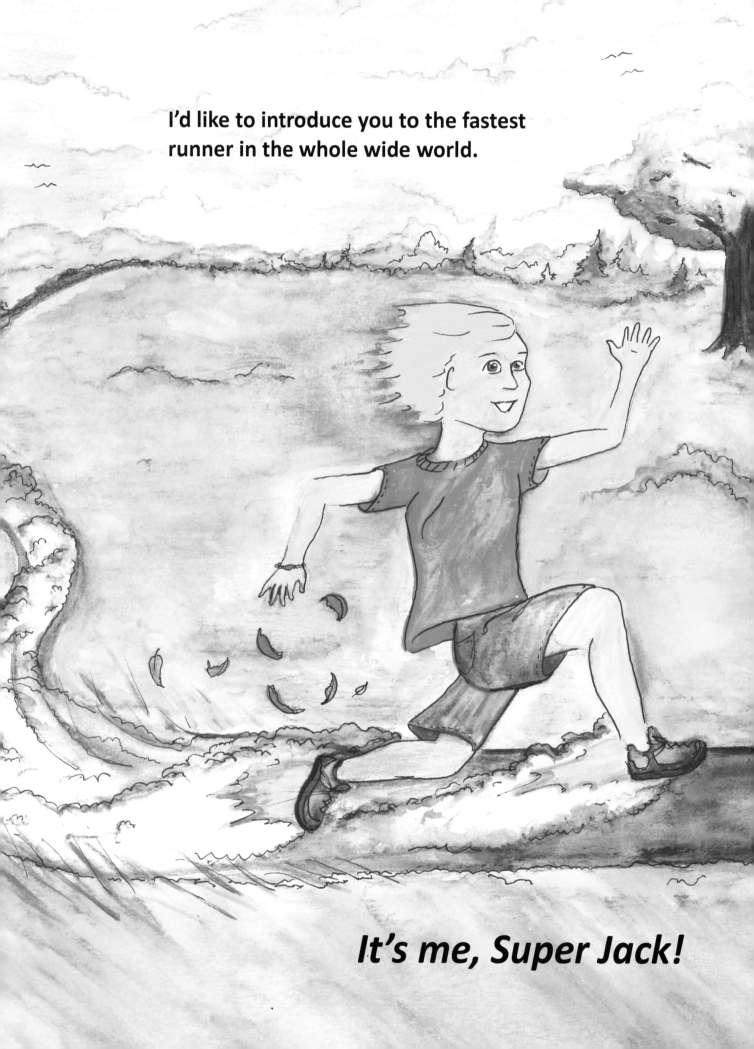

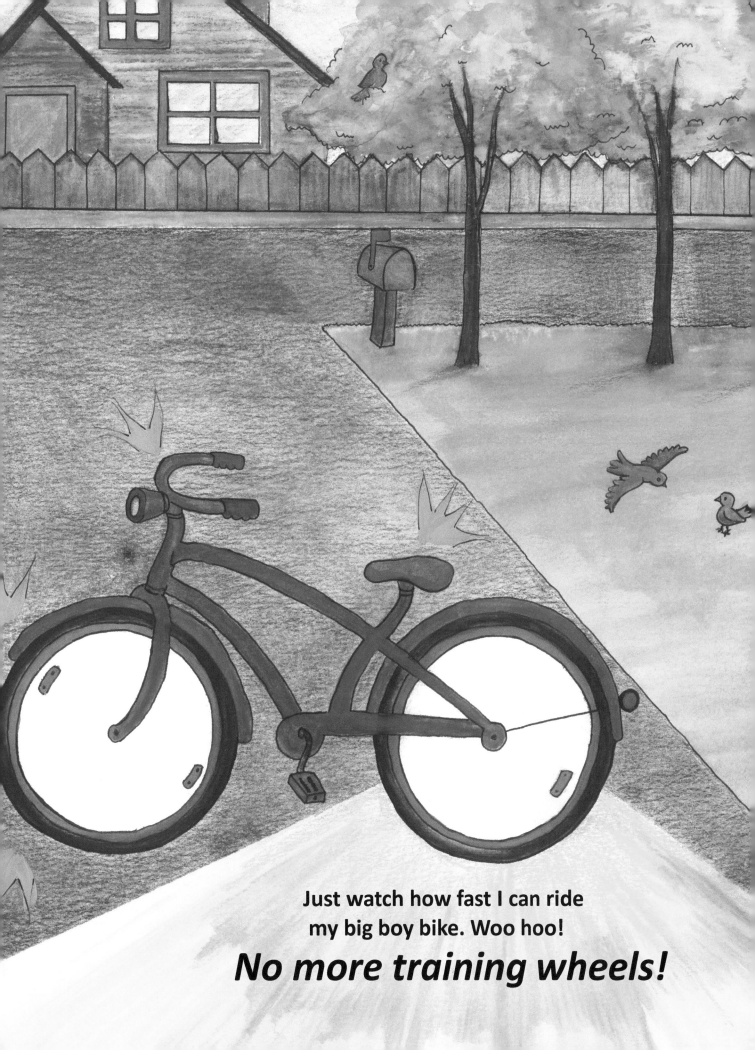

Just watch how fast I can ride
my big boy bike. Woo hoo!

No more training wheels!

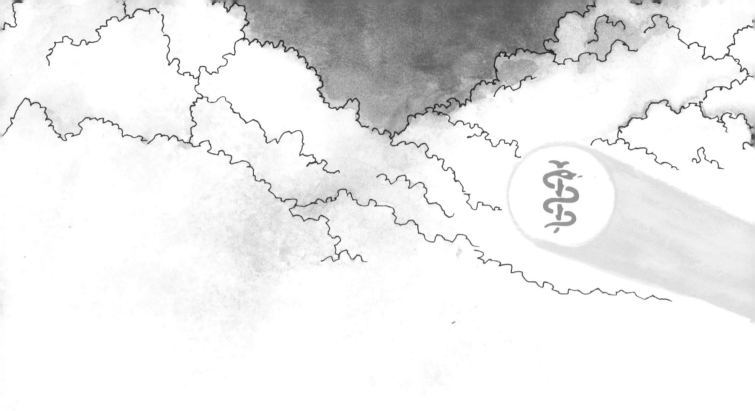

See my cool bracelet?

I like to pretend that it gives me super powers, but really I wear it because I have food allergies. I'm allergic to milk, eggs and peanuts. I wear my bracelet all the time...even in the bathtub.

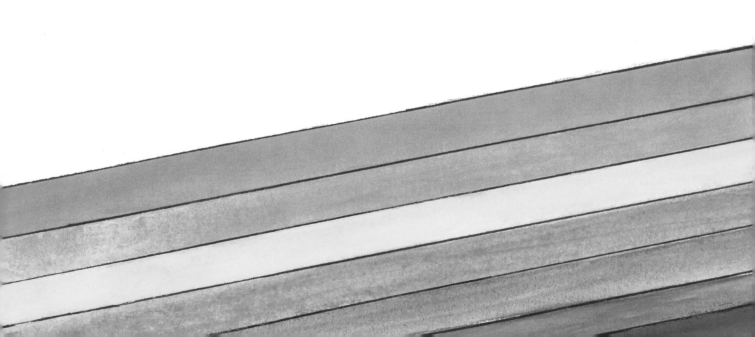

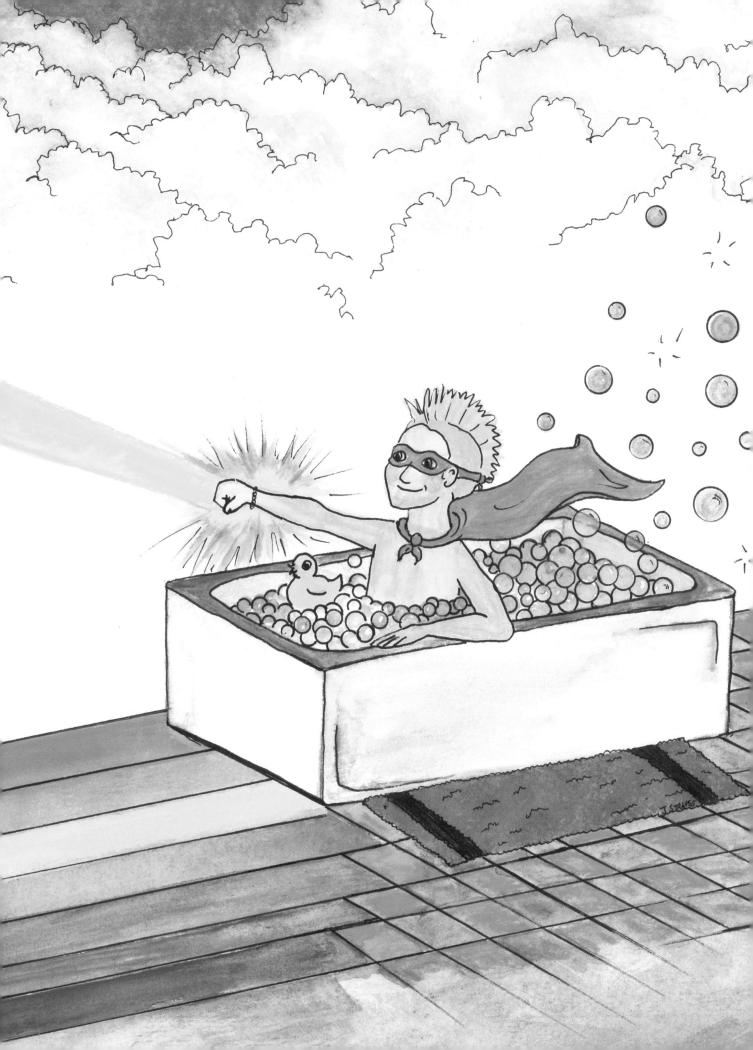

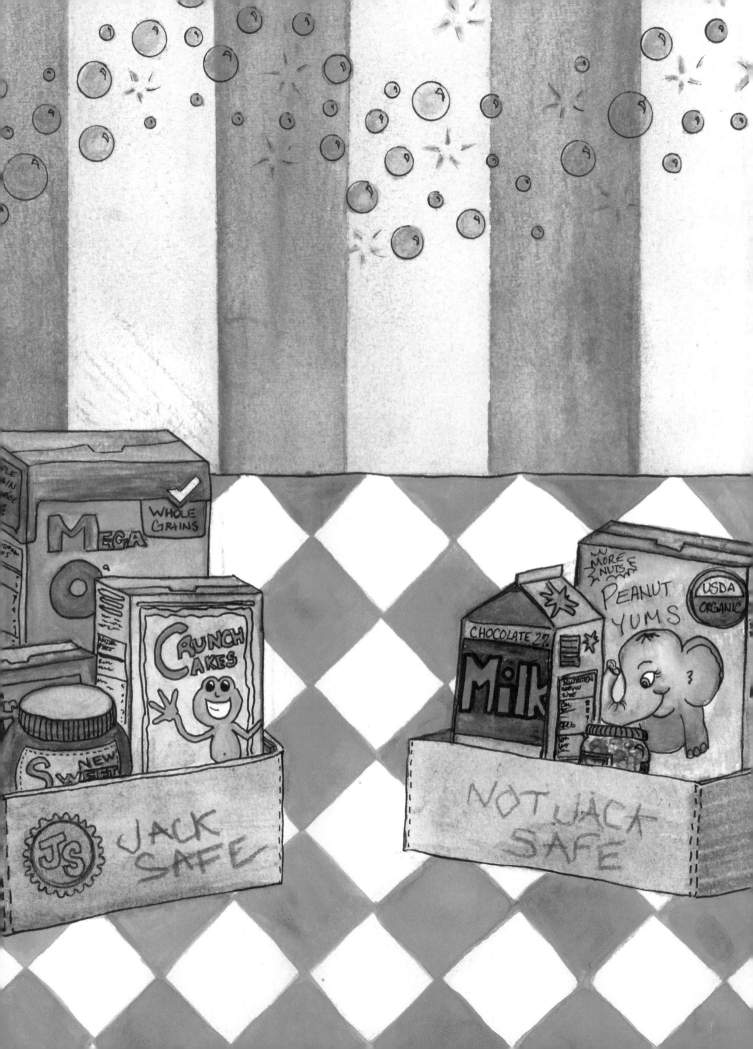

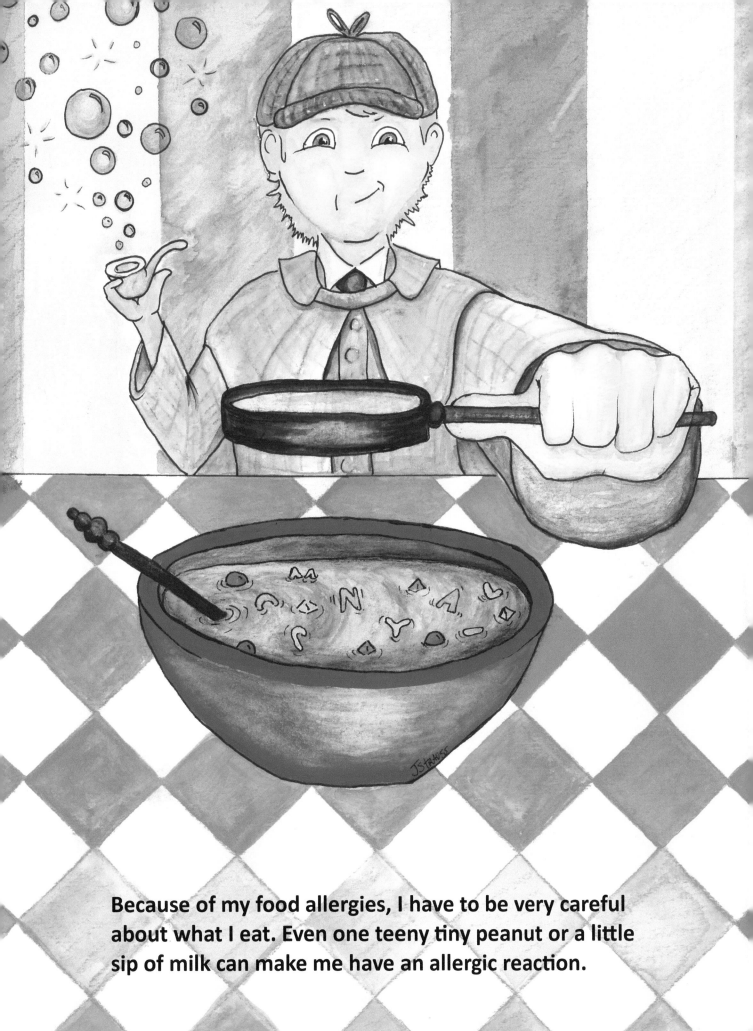

Because of my food allergies, I have to be very careful about what I eat. Even one teeny tiny peanut or a little sip of milk can make me have an allergic reaction.

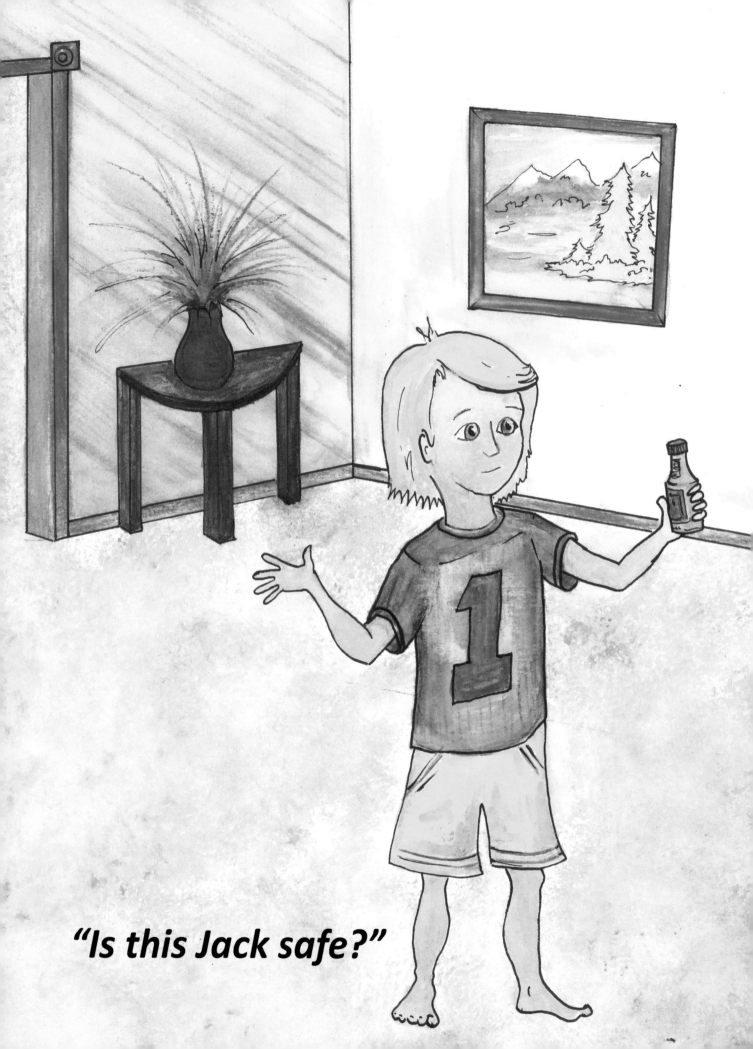

"Is this Jack safe?"

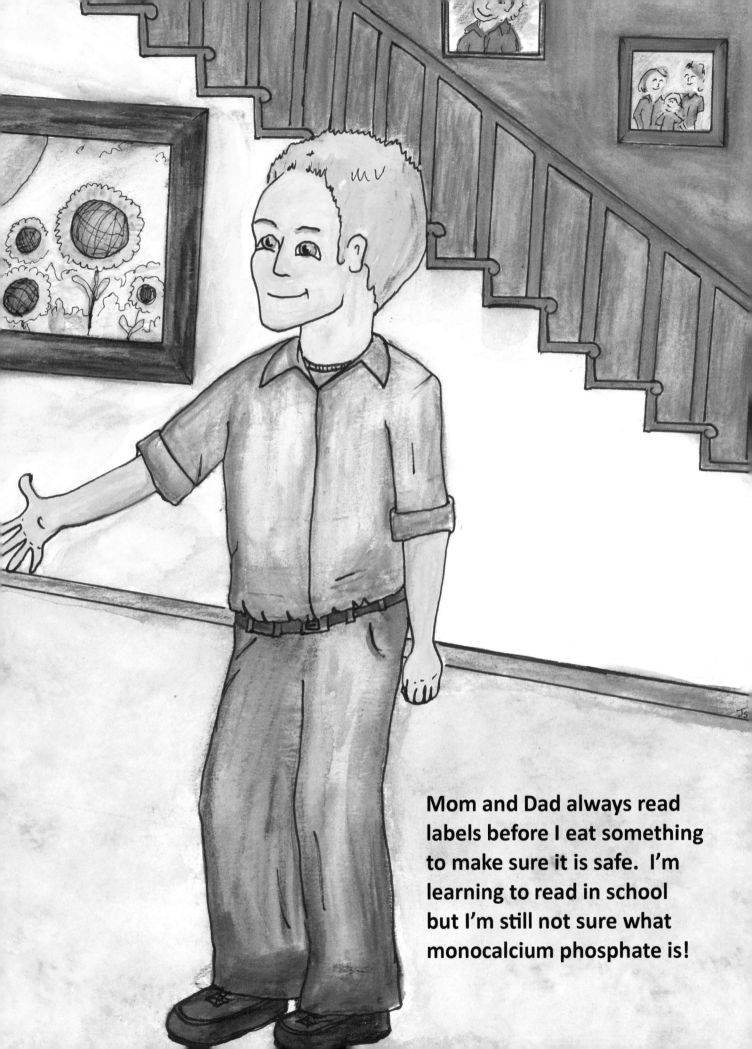

Mom and Dad always read labels before I eat something to make sure it is safe. I'm learning to read in school but I'm still not sure what monocalcium phosphate is!

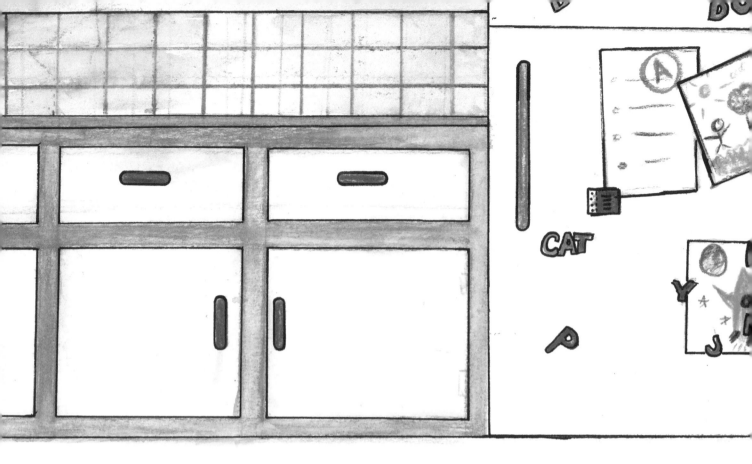

When I'm at home, Mom keeps my food on my very own shelf. She also puts

"*Jack Safe*"

stickers on everything so that our babysitter knows what I can eat.

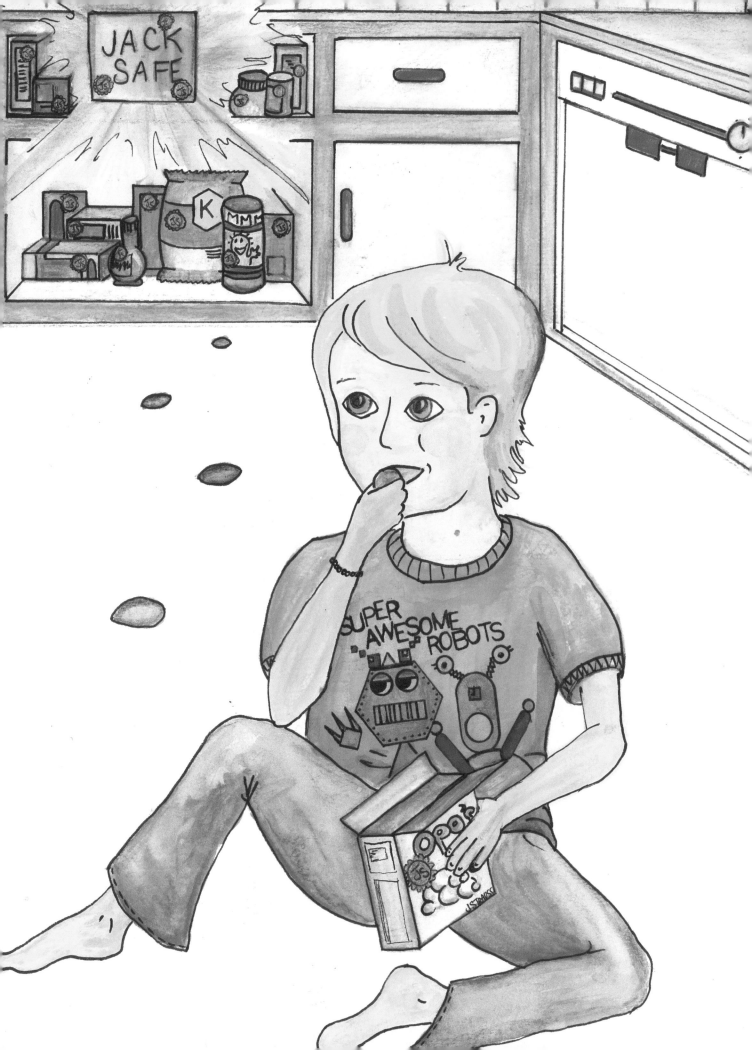

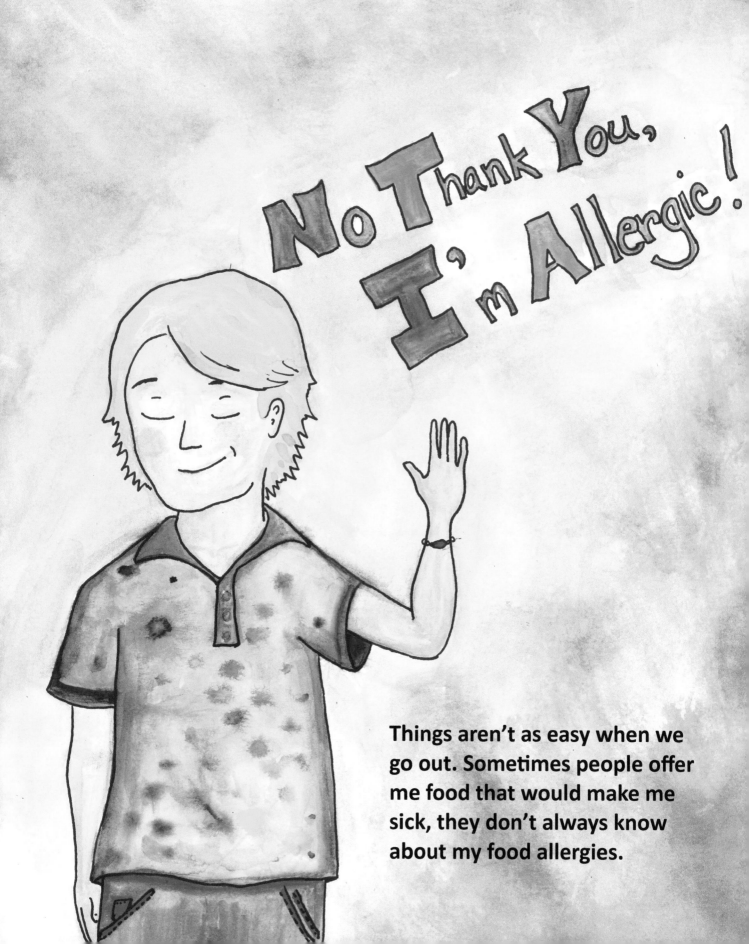

Things aren't as easy when we go out. Sometimes people offer me food that would make me sick, they don't always know about my food allergies.

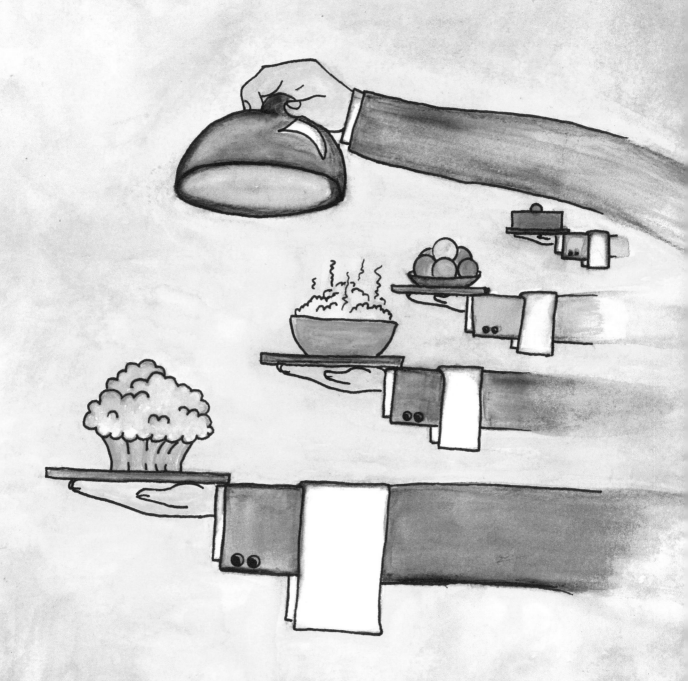

Mom and Dad say that when that happens
I should just smile and say,

"No thank you, I'm allergic".

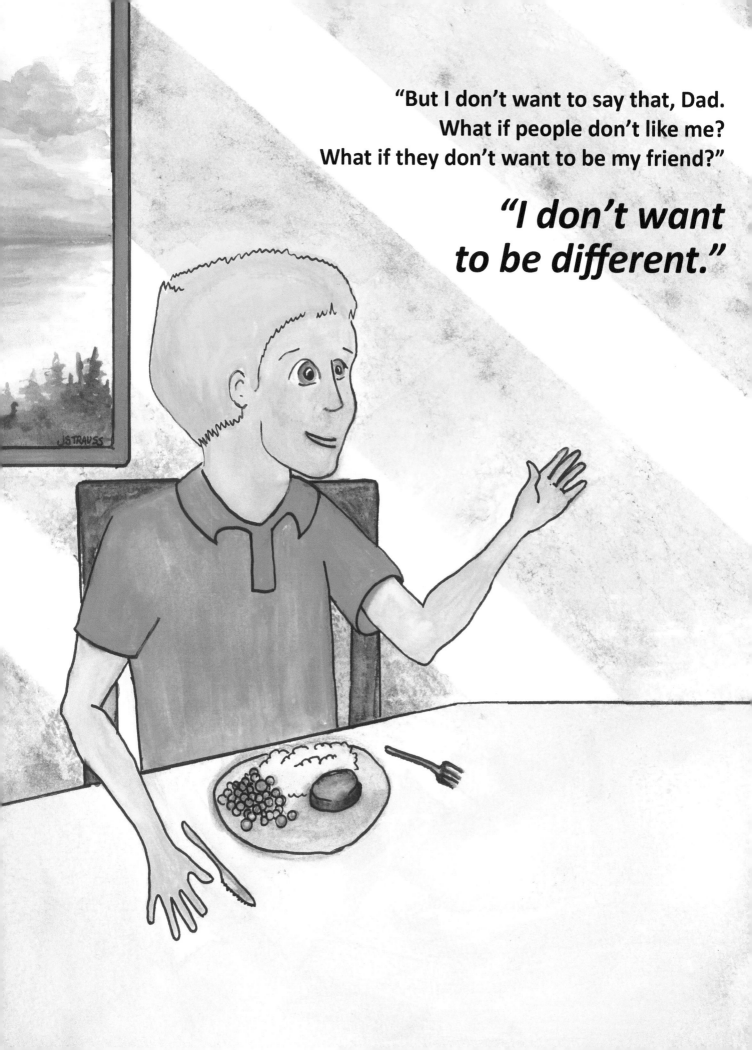

"Jack, everyone is different but that is not a bad thing."

"Yes, your food allergies make you unique, but so does your sense of humor and your smile. That's why people like you, that's why they want to be your friend!"

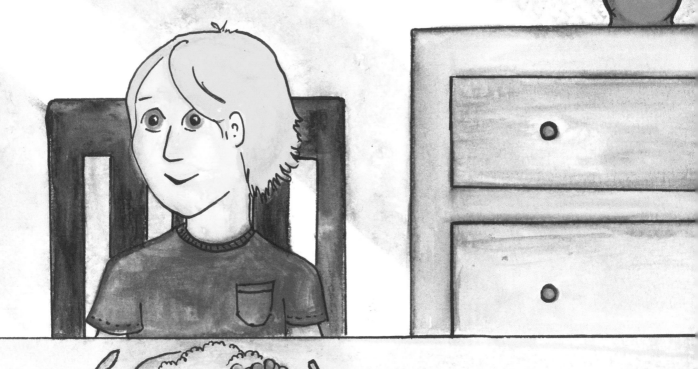

"And because I'm the fastest runner in the whole wide world?" I said. "Yes that too," laughed Dad.

I was still a little nervous but I promised Dad that I would try.

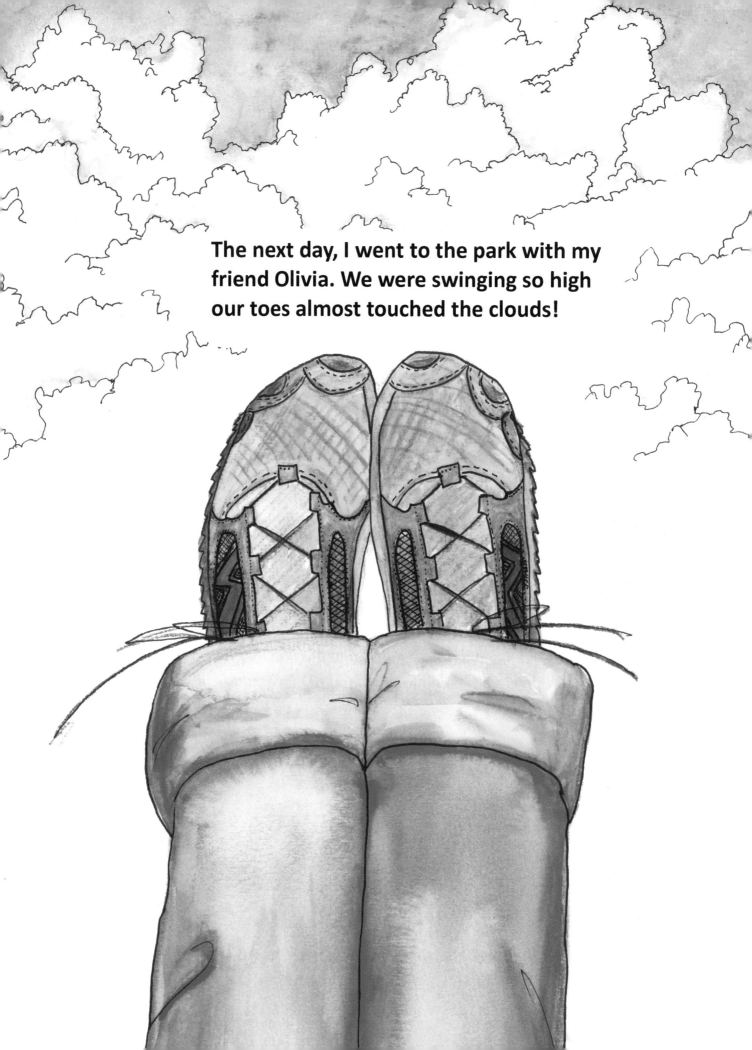

The next day, I went to the park with my friend Olivia. We were swinging so high our toes almost touched the clouds!

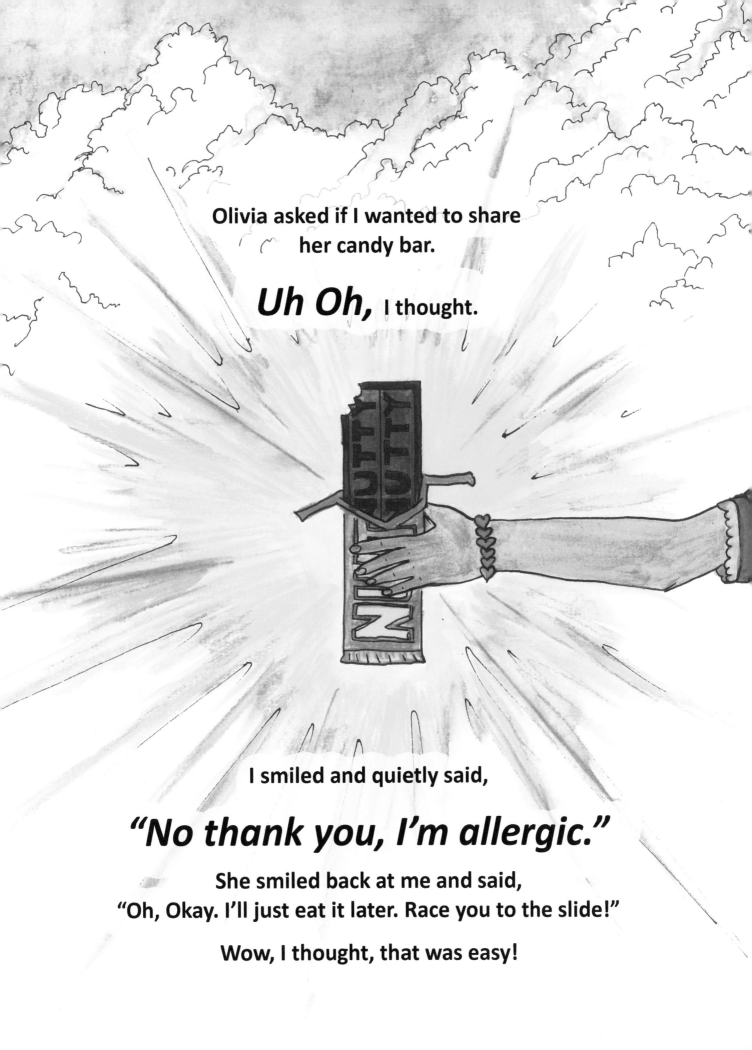

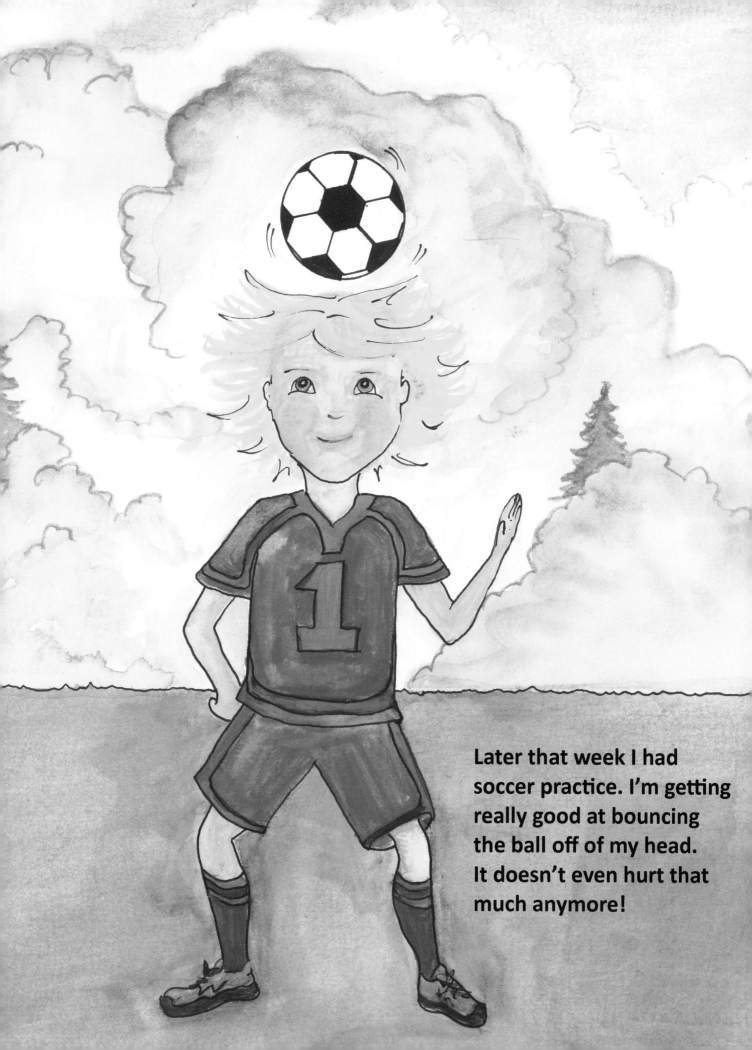

Later that week I had soccer practice. I'm getting really good at bouncing the ball off of my head. It doesn't even hurt that much anymore!

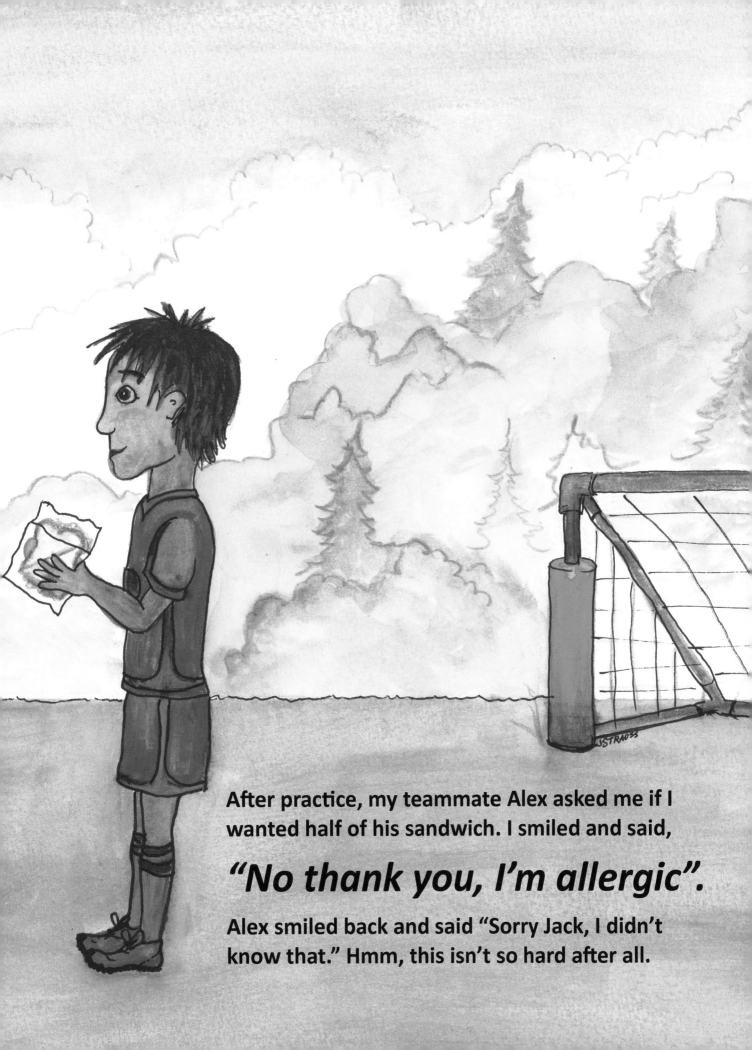

After practice, my teammate Alex asked me if I wanted half of his sandwich. I smiled and said,

"No thank you, I'm allergic".

Alex smiled back and said "Sorry Jack, I didn't know that." Hmm, this isn't so hard after all.

On Saturday I went to my friend Michael's birthday party. I was a little sad because I knew I wouldn't be able to eat the cake and ice cream like everyone else.

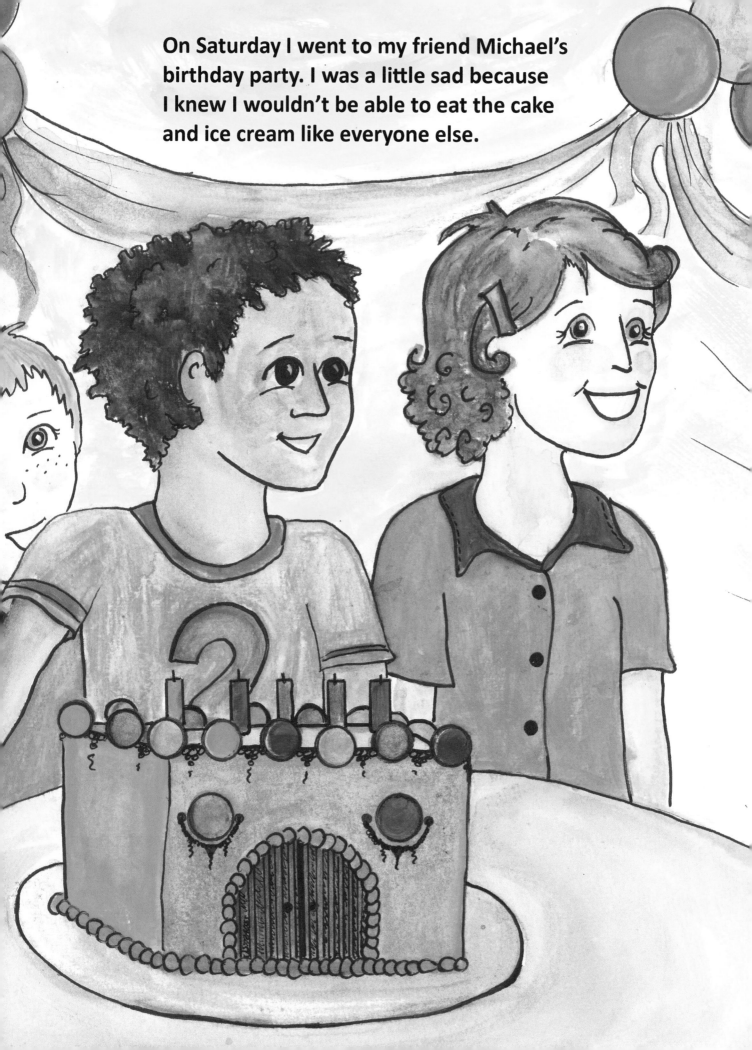

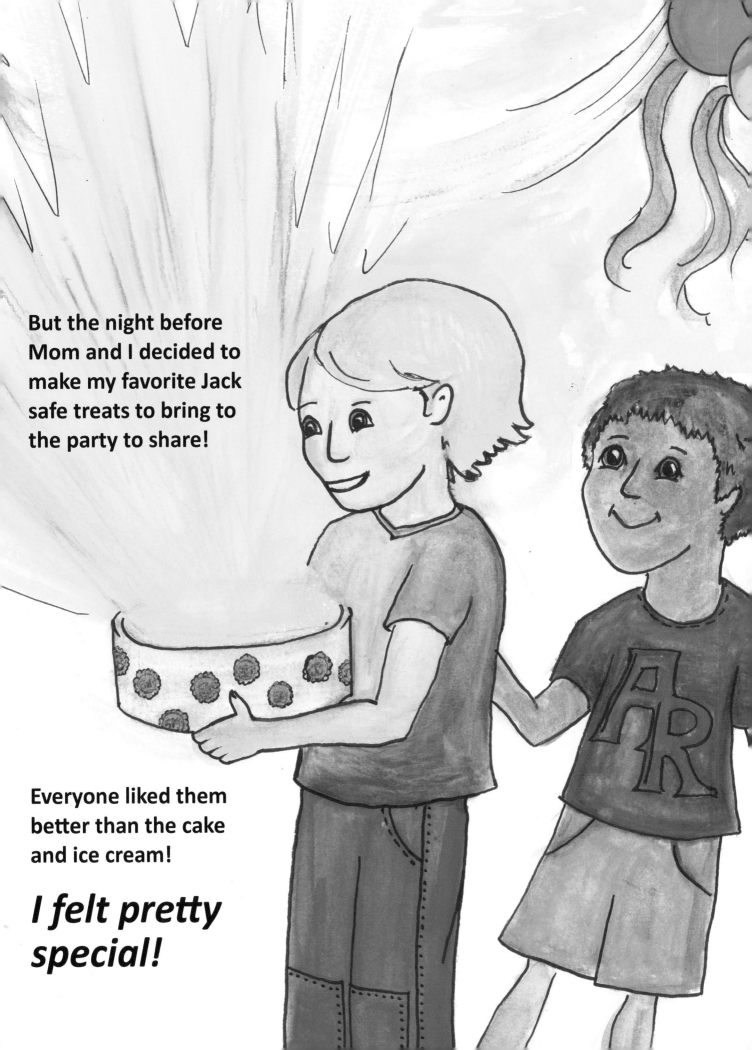

But the night before Mom and I decided to make my favorite Jack safe treats to bring to the party to share!

Everyone liked them better than the cake and ice cream!

I felt pretty special!

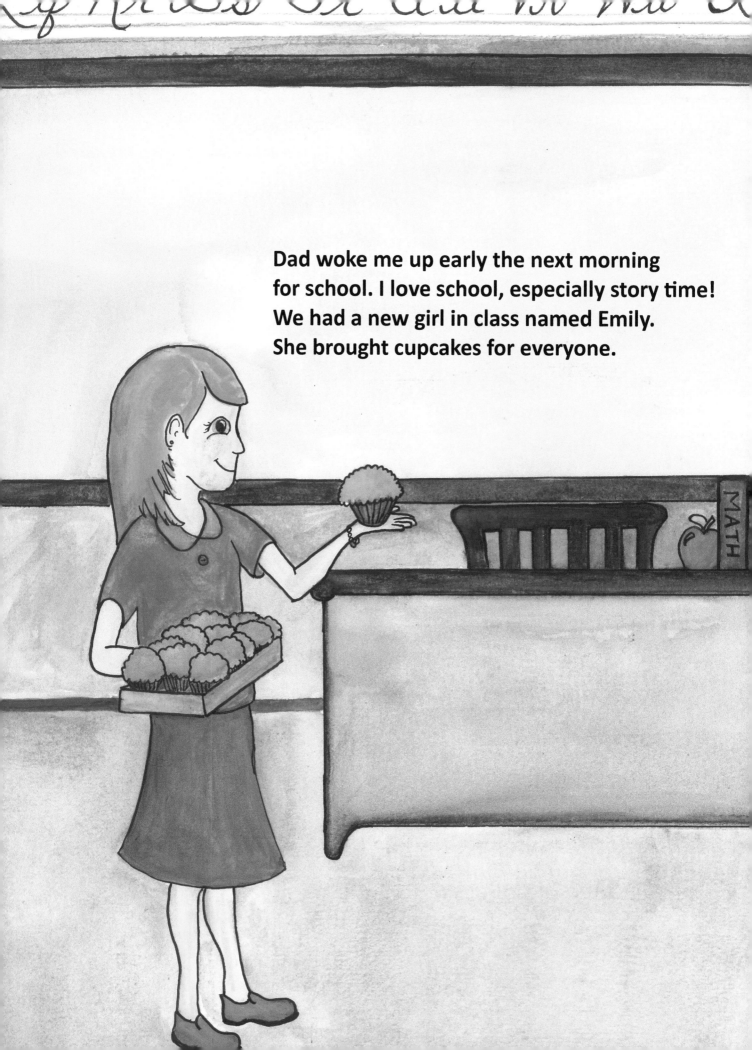

Dad woke me up early the next morning
for school. I love school, especially story time!
We had a new girl in class named Emily.
She brought cupcakes for everyone.

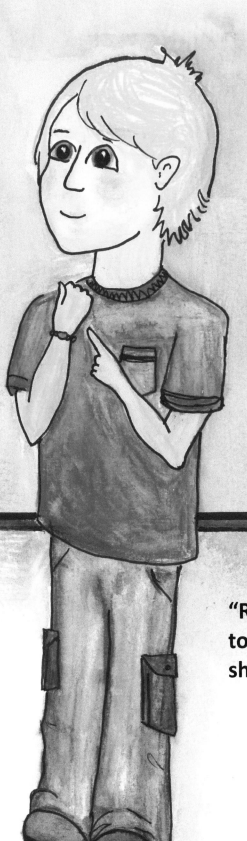

She asked me if I would like one and I smiled and said,

"No thank you, I'm allergic".

"Really?" She said. "I have allergies too. See my bracelet? I'm allergic to shellfish. Maybe we can be friends?"

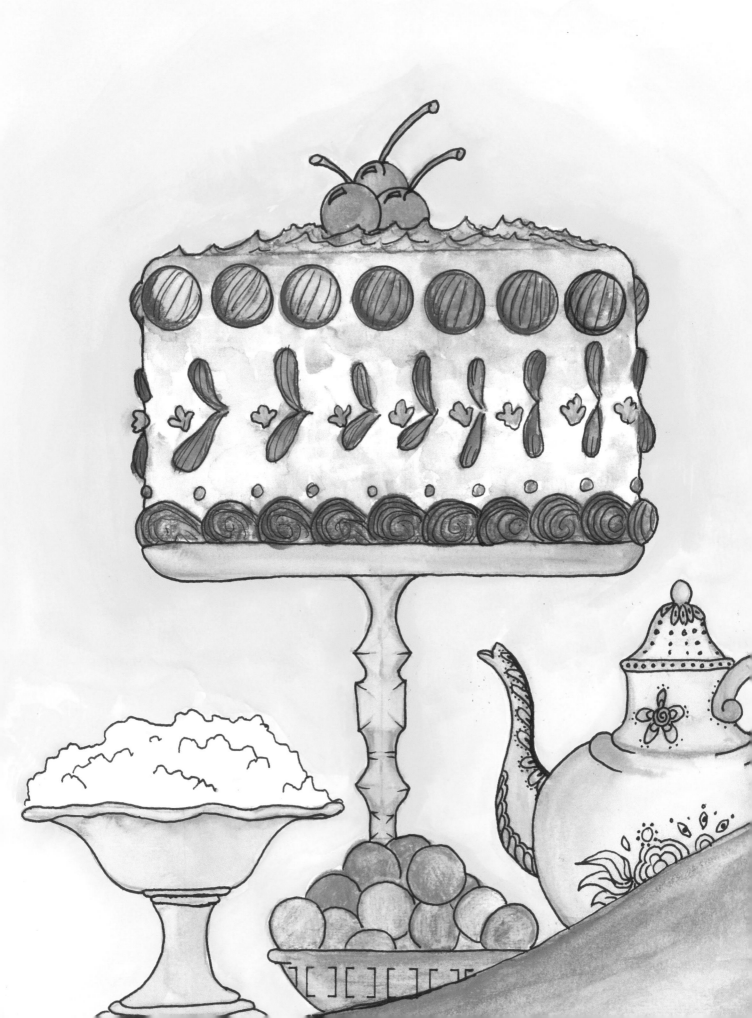

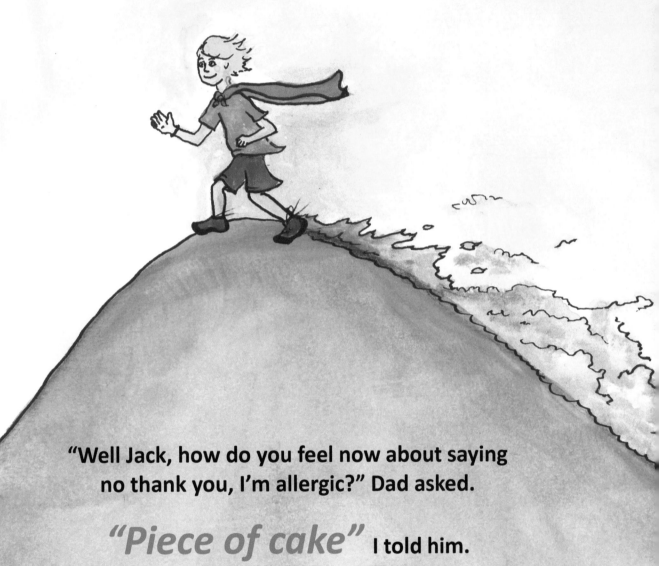

"Well Jack, how do you feel now about saying no thank you, I'm allergic?" Dad asked.

"Piece of cake" I told him.

"Make that a Jack safe piece of cake. No milk, no eggs and no peanuts."

CPSIA information can be obtained
at www.ICGtesting.com
Printed in the USA
LVHW070527100122
708178LV00012B/69